Intermittent Fasting For Women

Why Women Must Fast Differently Than Men

Hannah Golden

Table of Contents

reproduction of any of the following work, including precise information, will be considered an illegal act, irrespective whether it is done electronically or in print. The legality extends to creating a secondary or tertiary copy of the work or a recorded copy and is only allowed with the express written consent of the Publisher. All additional rights are reserved.

The information in the following pages is broadly considered to be a truthful and accurate account of facts, and as such any inattention, use or misuse of the information in question by the reader will render any resulting actions solely under their purview. There are no scenarios in which the publisher or the original author of this work can be in any fashion deemed liable for any hardship or damages that may befall them after undertaking information described herein.

Additionally, the information found on the

following pages is intended for informational purposes only and should thus be considered, universal. As befitting its nature, the information presented is without assurance regarding its continued validity or interim quality. Trademarks that mentioned are done without written consent and can in no way be considered an endorsement from the trademark holder.

Your FREE Intermittent Fasting Meal Plan

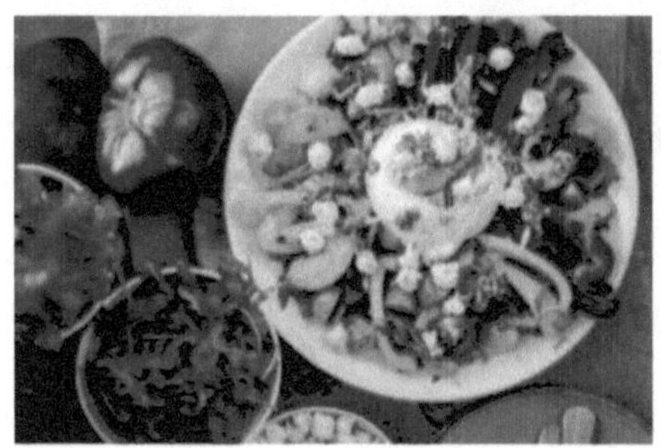

Subscribe to my email list and get your free IF meal plan and food guide. Learn what foods to avoid and what foods to stick to during time-restricted eating.

Visit:

HannahGoldenLifestyle.com/fastingmealplan

Introduction

Thanks for grabbing a copy of my book! Before we get started, let me introduce myself. My name is Hannah and I am a Yoga instructor, kickboxer and fitness enthusiast. I have tried many diets including vegan, vegetarian, Keto, Paleo and Intermittent Fasting.

Staying fit is a passion for many people, but dieting is the one thing that stops most of us in our tracks. See, it can be fun to go on hikes, hit the gym or play a sport. Yet avoiding donuts for the rest of your life isn't fun for anyone. Especially when you see your friends or significant other looking better than you and eating whatever they want! I have spent countless hours reading up on the latest diet trends. I have even tried a good number of them, only to give up weeks, months or even years in.

Let me tell you guys a little secret: not one diet is going to work for everyone.

I know, it sucks! If there was one diet that would just work, then we would have it all figured out by now. The truth is, diet is very complicated because everyone is so different. Each person has a unique genetic makeup in our DNA so we all respond differently to certain diets. For example, many people thrive on a plant-based, vegan diet. They can lose weight, feel good and keep that lifestyle up for years. I was determined to make a vegan diet work and kept it up for about three years. Then I had to stop because my iron levels were constantly too low.

Trust me, I tried everything to get my iron levels up. I ate all the iron-rich vegan foods, tried some supplements and everything. Eventually, I realized that my body was simply rejecting the plant-based iron and needed to get it through meat. I had to listen to my body, and you should always listen to yours.

This is why I decided to write a book on intermittent fasting specifically for women. To be perfectly honest, men have a much easier time fasting and they see the benefits (ie. more muscle mass, burning fat) a lot quicker than women.
If not done properly, intermittent fasting presents unique risks and side effects to women that don't happen to men.

For example, women respond differently to starvation than men. A woman is hardwired to keep a healthy weight and eat enough food because if she were to get pregnant, her body needs to support the baby. Cravings will be stronger for a woman and hormone balances will be thrown off. When a woman experiences starvation, her body sends a signal to the brain to stop releasing GnRH. This hormone is responsible for releasing two reproductive hormones (LH & FSH).

Since the body has stopped producing reproductive hormones, the ovaries will start to think that the woman is unable to support a healthy baby and so they act accordingly. They may stop ovulation, cause irregular periods or severe PMS. All side effects that a man would never have to worry about.

Intermittent fasting is one of the most promising new methods of weight loss and is proven to provide countless benefits for the body. It works wonders on your blood sugar, allows your body time to detox and allows you to build muscle mass and endurance without more exercise.

A woman can still see the positive effects of intermittent fasting but only if it is done correctly and tailored to fit the lifestyle and body of a woman. This book is going to show you how you can use intermittent fasting to reap the benefits while reducing the negative side effects if you are a woman.

What is Intermittent Fasting (IF)?

Intermittent fasting is not really a diet, it is a lifestyle. It is simply the act of taking a "break" from eating constantly and giving your body a chance to focus on other important tasks. Rather than avoiding certain foods or eating less in order to restrict calories, IF simply restricts the amount of time that you have to eat, thereby restricting calories and increasing the time your body has to burn fat and get rid of toxins.

If you manage to get your eating schedule down to a 16:8, that means that you are fasting for 18 hours and only eating within an 8-hour time frame. In those 8 hours, you will have only two or three meals. Since there is only so much food we can fit in our stomachs in one sitting, simply reducing the amount of time you spend eating will greatly reduce the overall amount of food that you eat.

In order to get the most benefits and results out of this lifestyle, it is best to pair it with a high-fat low carb diet, however, this is not absolutely necessary, and IF is very forgiving. If you practice fasting for 18 hours on most days, your body will allow for a cheat day every week and you will not see many negative side effects for doing so.

The Benefits of Intermittent Fasting

Now that I have scared you off IF with what it can do to your female body, let me tell you why it's still worth it and why I have adopted this diet into my life. There are many benefits of time restricted eating, or fasting and it is a very healthy way to live your life. Here is a breakdown of why adopting this lifestyle will benefit your health.

Weight Loss:

I am just going to get the obvious one out of the way. Intermittent fasting is a very easy way to lose weight and burn fat. Most of us eat a carb-filled breakfast in the morning (let's say around 7:00 am) and continue to snack and eat throughout the whole day, until about 8:00 or 9:00 pm. This means you're constantly providing your body with readily available energy, usually in the form of carbohydrates. Your body burns through carbs, then you eat a snack and your body burns more carbs from the snack you just ate. Then you have your next meal and the body burns *those* carbs. This cycle repeats throughout the whole day.

When does your body have time to burn excess fat? If you're constantly providing your body with readily available energy sources, it will simply use that and will not only avoid burning excess fat, it will store the extra fat for later! This is why it's so easy to gain weight on the regular high sugar, high carb diet while eating and snacking throughout the day.

When your body has a period of starvation or fasting, it gives it the time it needs to start burning excess fat and use that fat for energy instead of the carbs. Now, you don't have to avoid carbs all together but using intermittent fasting along with a low carb, high fat/protein diet will cause you to lose weight even faster! I'll go into this detail when discussing specific diets that you can pair with IF.

Increased Muscle Mass

Fasting allows for increased production of Human Growth Hormone (or HGH). Studies have shown that fasting for five days provides an increase of HGH by 300%! You don't need to fast for five days to reap the benefits though. Even fasting for a few hours at a time will significantly increase the presence of HGH in your system.

Normally, HGH is secreted into our blood system at night time. This is because our body is not concerned with digesting or processing food so it has the time to "rejuvenate" if you will. HGH is the hormone responsible for building and preserving muscle mass.

It makes total evolutionary sense why this would be the case. See when our ancestors were out hunting and gathering for food, they would be hit with winter, a time where there was less food and more starvation. In order to combat this starvation, human bodies would not start to use muscle mass in order to provide energy because that would put the person at a disadvantage if a lion or tiger came to attack them. Our muscles are the best line of defense and we need them to survive. So, our body will try its best to preserve our muscles in time of starvation. It much rather burn our useless fat!

Anti-Aging and Building of Body Tissue

When your body is not tied up with digesting and processing food, it has time to focus on detoxing and getting rid of "waste". This process is called autophagy. Autophagy is primarily motivated by Lysosome. Imagine lysosome like a magic wand that can turn waste into building blocks. In our bodies, building blocks are amino acids and they can have anti-aging properties, rebuild brain cells and rebuild important organ tissue such as for the heart, liver, and lungs.

When you fast, you allow autophagy to take place and so your body is completely rejuvenating itself. It is getting rid of waste and turning that waste into brand new healthy proteins and cells that will promote longevity and prevent disease.

Chapter 1: Why Women Should Fast Differently Than Men

When it comes to intermittent fasting, women often need to approach it differently than men. This is because a woman's reproductive system requires her body to react to starvation more severely than in males. This chapter will explore how the body reacts to fasting and starvation, the different reactions a woman's body has to fasting and starvation and the warning signs women should look out for when performing intermittent fasts. With the information provided here, you can best tailor your intermittent fasting to get the most benefit from it with the least amount of worry over the potentially negative effects.

What Fasting Does to the Body

The human body is a machine, and like all machines, it needs fuel through energy to continue to function. This energy is used to power two different types of functions; those that are part of the basal metabolic rate and those that are part of the physical activity level. The basal metabolic rate represents the background and automatic functions of the body. This includes all of the processes that keep a person alive, like the beating of the heart, breathing and brain function as well as the almost countless other processes that keep the human machine chugging. On the other hand, the physical activity level represents the energy needed for the body's movement.

The fuel the human body requires to provide its energy comes from food. While the body can get this energy from fats, carbohydrates, protein, alcohol or a combination of the four, normally, all of the cells of the body want to run on glucose. Glucose is the main energy source for almost every known organism. The body can break down most carbohydrates into glucose, though some, such as fructose, needs to be metabolized through the liver and converted into glycogen, a specific type of glucose. When the body has an abundance of glucose, it converts it into fatty acids that get stored in the fat or antipode cells for later use.

At times when the body has no glucose on hand to use as energy to power its cells, it turns to the glycogen stored in the liver as well as the smaller amounts stored in the muscles. This lack of glucose could be from either a diet extremely low in carbohydrates, such as Atkins and Keto or from fasting and starvation. Once the glycogen is low, the body turns to the stored fatty acids in the antipode cells and begins to cover them back into glucose.

At this point, the liver begins to release ketone bodies that tell most of the cells of the body to start using fatty acids for fuel while the brain continues to receive glucose from the converted fatty acids. Fueling the brain can take up to a quarter of the basal metabolic rate, and due to the blood-brain barrier, only glucose and ketone bodies can be used to fuel the brain. The blood-brain barrier protects the brain from blood-borne infections by limiting what the body allows into the brain.

As starvation progresses, the body starts to metabolize protein from the muscle cells into their component amino acids which the liver can convert to glucose to feed the brain. This is the point of fasting or starvation where a person would begin to lose muscle mass, but it can take a week or more of starvation to reach this point.

The exact timeline of these starvation processes will differ from person to person, but in general terms, it usually takes two to three days for the liver to start producing ketone bodies and begin the conversion of the fatty acids stored in the antipode cells into energy. Starvation mode, where the body starts to break down protein from the muscle tissues, begins four to five days after that.

For a modern person living with an abundance of readily available food, the way the body handles storing food energy in the antipode cells has led to a sharp rise in obesity but, in the distant and not so distant past, it has been an evolutionary bounty that enabled humanity to survive. Early humans existed as hunter/gatherers, getting all of their caloric intake from animals they could hunt and the wild growing fruits, vegetables and nuts that they could find in their environment. Having to survive periods of little food, such as when there were few big game animals to hunt or when the gathered plants were out of season, was a necessity.

To better enable survival through those lean periods with little food, the body stores what energy it doesn't immediately use to power itself as fat for later use. In starvation mode, the body ensures that the brain keeps getting as much energy as it needs through converting protein and fat into glucose because a well-fed brain will enable the person to best find the food needed to end the starvation cycle.

Fasting, Starvation, and Hormones

Fasting and starvation can have some drastic effects on a variety of hormones including sex hormones such as estrogen as well as hormones more related to metabolisms such as insulin and hunger-regulating hormones. Human growth hormones are also drastically affected by fasting and starvation.

Insulin is a hormone produced by the pancreas, and it promotes the absorption of glucose and other carbohydrates. In doing so, it functions to regulate the metabolism of fats and protein in addition to carbohydrates. The insulin level in the blood raises when food is consumed. With starvation and even short fasts, the insulin levels will drop significantly as there are no new carbohydrates from food for it to help absorb. This can result in lowering the chase of developing insulin resistance and type 2 diabetes. Additionally, it often leads to less water and salt retention in the kidneys and a loss in water weight. This is also a common side effect of a low carbohydrate diet.

Human growth hormone is created in the pituitary gland and has a large role in the development of the body during childhood and adolescents. Levels of it drop significantly as adults age. Human growth hormone has anti-aging as well as muscle building and fat burning effects that are still being studied. In short fasts, Human Growth Hormone levels have been observed rising significantly. Sometimes doubling or even rising 300% in 5-day fasts.

Hunger is regulated by two different hunger hormones; leptin and ghrelin. Leptin is an appetite suppressor that is created by fat cells and is thought to contribute to obesity through a person gaining resistance to its effect, leading them to eat even when leptin is telling their body they have enough. Leptin is found in greater amounts in the blood of obese people. Ghrelin performs the opposite, increasing the appetite. It is released by the stomach and signals the brain to eat more food. Ghrelin is found in lower amounts in obese people while it is found in greater amounts in those suffering from eating disorders such as anorexia.

Fasting and starvation have interesting effects on ghrelin that can actually lead to less hunger after a short fast. In studies where Ghrelin levels were checked every 20 minutes, it was found to be at its lowest at 9:00 in the morning. This seems counterintuitive as that is the time, for most people at least, when they have gone the longest without food. There is a reason breakfast contains the word break and fast.

The circadian rhythm likely has something to do with that. This is the body's internal clock that is mostly known for its regulation of the sleep cycle but also affects other bodily functions as a part of its sleep regulation. Suppressing the need to use the bathroom is an example of one of these other body functions that the circadian rhythm regulates. Suppressing the appetite as part of sleep prevents hunger from waking us too.

In addition to the counterintuitive lull in the early

morning, ghrelin levels were found to spontaneously peak and then recede three times a day. These peaks roughly coincide with lunch, dinner and the next day's breakfast, regardless of whether the food was consumed at the time or not. This shows that ghrelin has at least a partial learned component. The subjects of the research tended to eat three meals a day, and the ghrelin spikes tended to happen at their normal meal time.

After a twenty-four hour fast, ghrelin levels were found to remain relatively stable. Over a three day fast, ghrelin levels lowered each day, though they still peaked as a part of the circadian rhythm. Specifically, for women, there was good and bad news. They started and finished with higher levels of ghrelin compared to men, and their ghrelin levels spiked much higher than that of men during the fasts. This seems to show that women feel the effect of ghrelin much stronger than men. After a three day fast, however, the level of ghrelin in the women studied had dropped much steeper than in the men, so fasting might be more effective in lowering ghrelin in women than men. Overall, this study shows that short intermittent fasts do not cause persistent increases in ghrelin, meaning that, while hunger might increase during the fasting period, especially as you start intermittent fasting, it will not remain at high levels, and in fact will decrease.

Sex hormones, both male, and female can undergo significant changes in fasting and starvation. Due to the nature of a woman's reproductive system, this can have much greater effects on a woman's body compared to that of a man, and these effects are not limited to the reproductive system, so even women who are finished having children or do not intend to have children need to take care when performing intermittent fasting.

Sex hormones are released through a trio of different organs. The hypothalamus starts the process by releasing gonadotropin-releasing hormones. These travel through the body and reach the pituitary glands causing it to release both luteinizing and follicular simulation hormones. These hormones travel to the gonads (ovaries in women and testes in men) where they trigger the release of estrogen and progesterone in women and testosterone in men.

Estrogen and progesterone play an important part in the regulation of a woman's cycle including triggering the release of mature eggs in ovulation as well as supporting pregnancy. Testosterone production in the testes of men is partially responsible for the production of sperm. For men, studies of Muslim men fasting during Ramadan has shown that fasting can have a temporary effect on the production of sperm during the period after the fast, but this effect is minimal. The potential consequences for women can be much larger.

Due to the nature of a woman's cycle, the timing of the hypothalamus' release of gonadotropin-releasing hormones needs to occur right on schedule for everything to line up. Unfortunately, it can be ultra-sensitive to outside factors such as fasting. Even the missing of a single meal can put its timing off. As with the storage of fat, there are evolutionary reasons for this. Pregnancy takes a great deal of energy, and while some animals, such as some bears, can actually pause pregnancy when food is too scarce, the human body cannot do this. When the body is deprived of food, it thinks that there is not enough to support a pregnancy and disrupts the woman's cycle to prevent it.

If this were the only effect, fasting could be a miracle birth control method, but unfortunately, estrogen and other female hormones are deeply connected to the metabolic system as well. Estrogen receptors in the liver are dependent on amino acids to be activated. Once activated these trigger aspects of the reproductive cycle such as the thickening of the uterine wall. The amino acids are taken from consumed protein, so fasting or low protein diets can disrupt reproduction. Further, there are estrogen receptors all over the body where it takes part in regulating several functions such as bone formation, mood, cognition, and digestion.

Estrogen even plays a part in suppressing hunger, by stimulation of the production of peptides that function as appetite suppressors. The drop in estrogen levels common during and after menopause can lead to an increased appetite and weight gain. The drop in estrogen as part of a fast can possibly trigger an increased appetite.

Fasting is only one of the potential causes of a woman's cycle getting out of balance. Other causes can be due to the poor nutritious quality of their diet, illness or infection, inadequate sleep, over-exercising, and too much stress. All of these factors put extra stress on the body, making it decide that it would be a bad time for her to become pregnant.

How This Changes Intermittent Fasting for Women

As fasting can lower estrogen levels and estrogen is an important hormone for women's whole-body health, some care needs to be taken when deciding to start intermittent fasting. There are several different methods of intermittent fasting that will be discussed in the next chapter. Some of them provide a more gentle approach while others can be a bit harsh. To minimize the negative effects intermittent fasting can have on a woman, it is best to favor one of the less extreme methods of intermittent fasting and gradually increase the amounts or lengths of fasts to let the body adapt to the fasting regimen.

It is also vital that a woman pay attention to both her body and mind as she introduces her body to fasting. Several warning signs can signal you have gone too far with your intermittent fasting. If any of the following happen, either stop your intermittent fasting or if they manifest after you have increased the length or amount of fasts, return to less or smaller length fasts.

Irregularities in your menstrual cycle, or even having it stop can be a major warning sign. Insomnia, both in falling asleep or staying asleep can also be a warning sign. Pay attention to your skin and hair. If you develop more acne or dry skin, pull back, same if you begin to lose hair. A persistent feeling of always being too cold, as long as it is a new feeling, can also be cause for alarm.

Some of the mental side effects to look out for are mood swings as well as increased sensitivity to stress. A drop in your sex drive can also be cause for concern. If you exercise, pay attention to how well you recover from your workouts. If it starts to get longer, it might be time to cut back on fasts.

Women Who Shouldn't Fast

In addition to the warning signs that fasting could have too much effect on your estrogen levels, there are a couple of groups of women who should not attempt intermittent fasts or should undertake them with great caution.

Pregnant women shouldn't fast at all. Pregnancy requires a great deal of energy, and with human babies, the fetus comes first. This means that your body will see to the needs of the fetus over the needs of the mother. Fasting in pregnancy will cause a great deal more stress on a woman's body than fasting when not pregnant. This can lead to greater health issues for both mother and child and should be avoided.

Women who are trying to conceive should also avoid intermittent fasting. As we have discussed, fasting can have an effect on your reproductive hormones and will make you less fertile because your body will think you are starving and might not be able to support a baby.

Women who have a great deal of stress in their life already and those with sleeping issues should approach intermittent fasting with great caution. The extra level of stress caused by intermittent fasting's estrogen lowering tendency can exacerbate their existing stress-related issues.

Finally, women who have had issues with eating disorders in the past should be extra vigilant about intermittent fasting as it puts them at risk of a relapse.

Chapter 2: The Different Methods of Intermittent Fasting

Intermittent fasting can provide the health benefits of starvation mode or a severe calorie restrictive diet without the difficulty and muscle loss that come with prolonged fasts or extended periods of severely restricted calorie intake. Studies have shown that it can boost your metabolism, reverse insulin resistance and even prevent type 2 diabetes, and improve heart health. Animal studies have also shown that it can lead to a longer life.

Several different forms of intermittent fasting can often be done concurrently. Some of these are more extreme than others, and all of the different types have their pros and cons. This chapter will explore several different intermittent fasting methods, discussing both the pros and cons and how they can be used together. This will touch on the type of diet that works best with intermittent fasting as well as how to approach starting intermittent fasting, though both of those topics will be covered in a more thorough nature in the following chapters

Preparing to Fast

Just flipping a switch and deciding to start intermittent fasting can work, but it can also add unnecessary stress to your body, and as we covered in the last chapter, women's bodies are already more sensitive to diet changes than men's, adding extra stress should be avoided. Shifting your diet into one that has a low intake of carbohydrates with high intake of proteins and healthy fats can make intermittent fasting more effective. Weaning yourself off of drinks that contain sugar or artificial sweeteners before a fast can make it easier as well.

During the fasting periods of your intermittent fasting regimen, staying hydrated is important, but your choice of drinks needs to be calorie free. Water, unsweetened tea and black coffee are ideal for this, but diet sodas and other drinks that contain artificial sweeteners might not be ideal. This is an area of current research, but there have been some findings that show that, while artificial sweeteners have no calories, they can spike insulin levels by basically tricking the body into thinking they contain sugar. With intermittent fasting, one of the benefits is the lowering of insulin levels. Spiking your insulin levels, even without the presence of sugar, could counteract this benefit.

Another issue with artificial sweeteners is that they can leave you with an expanded craving for sweets. During fasting periods, this can lead to greater temptation to break the fast with a sweet treat. It can also lead to overindulgence of sweets when the fasting period has ended. Some proponents of intermittent fasting claim that one does not need to worry about what you eat when not on a fast. There might be a nugget of truth to that idea when using intermittent fasting for its health benefits and weight management, but for weight loss, overindulgence after a fast can be problematic. Binge eating is almost never a good idea, regardless.

A habit of drinking diet sodas can be tough to break, therefore weaning yourself off before you start intermittent fasting will make it easier to stay with it. For those who prefer a little taste to their water, adding a packet of crystallized lemon or lime to your water or a small amount of unsweetened lemon juice can add a touch of flavors with minimal calories. For example, lemon juice only has 7 calories per oz. Some people prefer the bubbles of carbonated water, and they can drink club soda or seltzer. Be sure to stay away from tonic water as it contains sugar.

Intermittent fasting works for weight loss by using the body's fat stores for energy instead of converting food into readily available energy. This works along the same lines as low carb diets such as Atkins, South Beach, and Keto. These diets all work in the same fashion and require modifying your diet to minimize carbohydrates, while eating more protein and healthy fats to increase the burning of excess fat.

Diet and meal plans will be covered in the following chapters, and although modifying your diet towards low carbohydrate intake is not required, it can really help. At the very least, minimizing more processed carbohydrates such as sugars, white bread and rice will help to keep insulin spikes at bay, providing you the most benefits from your intermittent fasting.

The Glycemic Index can be an important tool to assist you in choosing the right foods. The Glycemic index documents the effects each food has on a person's blood glucose or sugar level. A 100 on the Glycemic Index is the equivalent of pure glucose. Foods that are low on the glycemic index, such as most beans, seeds, nuts and vegetables; cause the blood sugar level to rise slowly and steadily. On the other hand, high glycemic index foods, such as; white bread, white rice and high fructose corn syrup can cause the blood sugar levels to rise quickly as the body can break them down much faster. This leads to insulin spikes and can help to undo some of the benefits that intermittent fasting can provide.

One last thing before moving on to the different intermittent fasting methods is the type of foods to eat on fasting days. Many of the different intermittent fasting methods do not contain actual fasts, but instead, feature days where calorie content is severely restricted. The choice of foods to eat on these days can make the difference between success and failure. Low-calorie vegetables, soups, and lean proteins can offer the most feeling of fullness with the least amount of calories. When you are only consuming 500 calories on a particular day, they will fill you up much more than a pint of ice cream. Additionally, they will not lead to insulin spikes that could jeopardize the benefits of the intermittent fast.

16:8 Method

One of the most common, and easiest to adapt, methods of intermittent fasting is the 16:8 method. The ratio represents fasting hours to eating hours. When using the 16:8 method, you will fast for 16 hours of the day while eating during the other 8 hours. As most people sleep 7-8 hours, this method only requires fasting for about 8 hours of waking time.

When it comes to the 16:8 method, the exact eating window is up to the faster herself. For women who generally skip breakfast, a 12-8 window can work perfectly allowing them to eat lunch and dinner as they normally would, as long as they avoid night time snacking. Some women might prefer a 7-3 window allowing for a big breakfast and either a late lunch or a lunch and afternoon snack. If this works for you, stick with it but for many women, this can lead to too much craving in the late afternoon and evening.

One of the benefits of the 16:8 method of intermittent fasting is that it can easily be done every day. This makes it much more likely to become a habit, enabling it to be easier to follow. For those new to intermittent fasting, easing into it by trying a 16:8 fast for two to three days in a week can be the gentlest way to start intermittent fasting.

If it works for you, expanding it to every day can be the next step.

Most proponents of the 16:8 offer no limitations to the amount or types of exercises that can be done concurrently with the fasting periods. This is because the fast period in the 16:8 method is so small. Make sure to remain hydrated and look out for any of the warning signs I outlined at the end of the first chapter. If you get dizzy or lightheaded during exercise while in a fasting period, it is likely best to slow down or move your exercise period to the hours that you are eating, if possible. As your body gets more used to intermittent fasting, you will likely be able to perfume more strenuous exercises, even in fasting periods, but going slow to start is often best.

14:10 Method

The 14:10 method of intermittent fasting is an even gentler version of the 16:8 method. Unsurprisingly, instead of 16 hours of fasting to 8 hours when eating is allowed, in 14:10 the fasting period is 14 hours while you are allowed to eat for a 10-hour period. This method will likely provide less benefit than the 16:8 method for most people, but as the eating period is longer, it can be perfect for an introduction or for those that a more severe method of intermittent fasting is too much. It can also be combined with an occasional single day fast to provide the benefits of a longer fast in a more approachable way.

5:2 Method

Most of the intermittent fast methods could use better names, they sure love ratios, but with the 5:2 method, the ratio is not hours, but instead days. In the 5:2 method you eat normally five days of the week but eat an extremely reduced amount of calories on the other two days. Generally, this is twenty-five percent of your normal daily requirements or about 500 calories for women and 600 calories for men. Most of the proponents of the 5:2 method advocate splitting the fast days so that at least one non-fast day is scheduled between the fasts. It is easier to get through the fast days this way, and there is much less strain on the body when the fast days are not bunched together.

The calorie numbers here are general, the fast will not fail if you have 501 calories. Use them as guidelines and not hard and fast rules. Don't fret if you are over by even a few hundred calories. Often, when people are dieting, and they miss a restricted calorie number, they give up for the day and make it a cheat day. This occurs less likely when the calorie restriction is general and not specific. Furthermore, one of the benefits of intermittent fasting is that the days you are not fasting, or the times of the day you are not fasting, are kind of cheat days already, within reason so you can beat the craving simply by postponing it to the next time you eat normally.

During the fast days, staying hydrated is incredibly important. Hot beverages often help with hunger, and there are several savory broths or soups with few calories. If you are a fan of sushi, several brands of instant miso soup can be found in Asian groceries with under 20 calories a serving. Just watch out for the salt content. Lean proteins and low-calorie vegetables make for excellent eating on fast days with the 5:2 method. These offer the most filling options for so few calories. Herbs and spices can also be used to add a punch of low to no calorie flavor to make this food more exciting.

When using the 5:2 method for weight loss, make sure that you do not binge on your off days. Intermittent fasting can be a miraculous tool for weight loss and health improvement, but you will still need to generally eat well on your non-fasting days, ideally with a diet low in carbohydrates.

When starting a 5:2 intermittent fast, it is acceptable to ease into it. This can be done in one of two ways, or a combination of both. The first way to way to ease into it is to start with fast days that include more calories. For example, in the first week, limit your fast day calories to 1000 instead of 500. Lower this level to 750 the next week, or when you feel comfortable with the change, and finally move down to the 500-calorie level. Another method would be to start a 16:8 fast for a few days a week. After a couple of weeks of this, switch one of those

16:8 days with a 5:2 fast day. Add more 16:8 days as you get more used to it and, finally, switch another day to a 5:2 fast day. Combining both can lead to greater benefits, but it could also lead to some of the problems discussed in the first chapter. Should that occur, pull back on your fasting days.

At the start of a 5:2 fast it is usually better to limit the amount and type of exercise you perform during the fast days. Stick with a lower impact type of exercises like yoga or resistance training. Avoid cardio and heavy lifting as too much exercise during the beginning of intermittent fasting can cause extra stress to the body and also trigger strong feelings of hunger. As you progress, pay attention to what your body is telling you and use that information to move or change the amount and type of exercise you perform on fast days.

Alternate Day Fasting

This method uses the same fasting rules from the 5:2 method, roughly 500 calories on fasting days, but increases the number of fast days to every other day. This can be a powerful method of intermittent fasting, but it is certainly not for everyone and definitely not for beginners. It is ideal for low carb diets as it easily keeps you in ketoses. Use this method if you have been using the 5:2 method for a while and want to extend it.

Like the 5:2 method, this can be modified to make it easier to manage. For example, instead of 500 calories every other day, you could modify it so that every other fast day is only a half fast so: Monday, eat normally; Tuesday, 500 calories; Wednesday, eat normally; Thursday, 1000 calories, etc. This can make the alternate day fasts more manageable. One of the other issues with the alternate day fast is the consumption of alcohol. It is best to avoid alcohol on fast days and the alternate day fasts will eventually line up on a Friday or Saturday, the nights where the consumption of alcohol tends to be highest. Should you desire to drink on a fast day, it is best to skip the fast that day, but don't make it a habit.

Eat Stop Eat Method

This is the first method that contains an actual 24 hour fast. With the Eat Stop Eat method, you generally stop eating at six or seven in the evening and then fast until six or seven in the evening on the next day. This is repeated as much as once a week, but no more than that, especially for beginners. A full 24 hour fast can provide a lot of benefits, but it is not for everyone. Some will get headaches or dizziness from such a fast. Irritability is also a common issue.

If you decide to try the Eat Stop Eat method, only do so if you have some experience with the easier intermittent fasts and end it if you must. As with other fasts, make sure to keep hydrated.

Warrior Diet

The Warrior Diet, so named as it is an attempt to mimic the diet of our Paleolithic ancestors, is a more extreme version of the 16:8 method, using a 20:4 ratio with 20 hours of fasting and 4 hours of feasting in the evening. The thinking behind this diet is related to the paleo diet that tries to limit the types of food eaten to those that hunter-gatherer tribes would have had access to. This includes meats and fats as well as nuts, berries, and some vegetables. Excluded are grains and cereals as they were a product of agriculture. Dairy is also usually excluded, though not by all. Dairy rose with agriculture, so it was not a common food for hunter-gatherers.

The hunters, in those early hunter-gatherer groups, would spend their days hunting and then eat what they caught at night when they returned to camp. Al least that was the logic behind this fasting regimen. In reality, these groups could have eaten during the day as well. We can see this by studying more recent hunter-gatherer societies and their eating habits. Take the plains native Americans for example. Their primary hunting animal was the buffalo, and they would preserve the meat by making pemmican, basically a mixture of dried meat and fruit, rendered fat, nuts and honey. Pemmican kept for a long time and could provide sustenance for hunters while on the hunt.

Another problem with the thinking behind the Warrior Diet is that it only focuses on half of the hunter-gatherer dynamic, ignoring the gathering aspect. Most hunter-gatherer groups divided the labor by gender with men doing the majority of the hunting while the women and children gathered nuts, berries, fruits, and other plants closer to the home. Even if the men brought the meat home at night, the women and children likely munched on fruit or nuts during the day. Most proponents allow for a little munching of fruit or nuts during the day on the Warrior Diet.

There has been little research on the Warrior diet, but for followers of a paleo diet, it might be an interesting method of intermittent fasting, though obviously not for everyone.

Meal Skipping Method

Overall, one of the easiest methods of intermittent fasting is meal skipping. To get the most out of this method, it is best used in addition to an intermittent fasting regimen that includes at least a couple of 16:8 days a week or with the 5:2 method. The basics are to listen and understand the hunger signals of your body. Often, we confuse boredom or habit of actual hunger and eat when we really do not need to. This is an unforeseen consequence of living in a time of food bounty. With processed food, we have better access to high calorie, easily accessed glucose, than the people of any other time before us. This has enabled many of us to have never felt the pang of true hunger.

Through intermittent fasting, this changes and that enables the intermittent faster to better understand the signals her body is giving her. Once you know your body's signals, you will know when you are truly hungry or if you just want to eat out of habit. With that knowledge, you can skip the meals for which you are not hungry.

Chapter 3: Finding the Right Intermittent Fast to Fit Your Life

One of the main difficulties in sticking to a diet program is fitting its requirements into your life in general. While every woman's life is different, most of us lead hectic lives with limited time for meal prep and exercise. Given the great variety of different intermittent fasting methods, however, it is possible to tailor a personal intermittent fasting regime that will fit in with your already hectic life while providing the powerful benefits that intermittent fasting can provide.

This chapter will explore how to fit intermittent fasting into your life. This will include a brief look at mixing the different methods of intermittent fasting to both maximize their benefit while keeping the potential difficulties some women can have with them and to better adapt them to your lifestyle. It will also look at several different specific types of women and offer tips for women living a similar lifestyle on how intermittent fasting can work for them.

Finding the Best Fast for Your Life

The hard truth is that not every type of intermittent fast will work for every person. We have already covered some of the specific issues that women in particular face when it comes to intermittent fasting. Some women will find what they need with certain methods while others, trying the same type of intermittent fasting, will be overcome with temptation or cravings and be unable to complete it.

Experimentation with different methods, starting slow and adjusting your diet before fasting can be helpful when it comes to an intermittent fasting failure. One of the ways intermittent fasting helps you lose weight is to push the body to begin using the fatty acids stored in the fat cells for most of its fuel. Reducing the number of carbohydrates in your diet before fasting will likely provide more of this fat burning benefit by limiting the amount of glucose added to the body through eating.

For some, this can mean following a low carb diet though for others, eliminating the simple carbohydrates, such as sugars and white flours, by either reducing their use or substituting them for more complex carbohydrates, like whole grains can be good enough. Complex carbohydrates offer other benefits for intermittent fasters as they have a larger amount of fiber which can add a feeling of fullness their simpler cousins cannot.

Many proponents of intermittent fasting put little to no importance into what the faster eats during their eating window and this can work for some. If you try an intermittent fasting method without following a specific diet and find that it is not providing the weight loss you expected, modifying your diet can help.

Intermittent fasting can allow for a less extreme elimination of carbs while providing the same benefits. If you start from the position of not modifying the types of foods you eat during your non-fasting windows, start with the elimination of sugar. Continue with you chosen fasting methods for another two weeks while avoiding as much sugar as you can. If that is insufficient, move to reduce the amount of simple carbohydrates. If you are a bread lover, substitute white bread with whole grain. For pasta lovers, switching to whole wheat pasta or those made from other grains such as quinoa can help. Quinoa can be a wonderful substitute for rice, or you can try the low carb trick of making cauliflower rice. If you are still not getting the weight loss benefit from your intermittent fast at this point, switching to a low carb diet might provide it. Low carb diets and intermittent fasting will be covered in the next chapter.

Modifying your chosen intermittent diet method is another way to make sure that you are getting the most out of your intermittent fasts and fitting them into your lifestyle. Here, again, the importance of starting slowly cannot be overemphasized. Jumping into one of the more extreme methods of intermittent fasting will be more difficult to maintain and be much harder on the body, potentially leading to some of the negative effects that fasting can have on some women. Start with a 14:10 or 16:8 on two or three days a week and maintain this for a few weeks.

At this point, if the short daily fasts are not providing the weight loss benefits you desire, add a few more days of 14:10 or 16:8 to your routine or add a 500-calorie fasting day. After a few more weeks of this, you can maybe add another fasting day for a 5:2 method while keeping to the 14:10 or 16:8 on the other days. By ramping up the changes slowly, you will minimize the potential negative consequences, and your body will adapt to its new feeding schedule over the course of time.

Intermittent Fasting for Women That Want Children

Studies on the specific effects that intermittent fasting have on the reproductive system are ongoing, but there have been some alarming results in animal studies on female fertility. Because of these findings, it is best for women who want to have children in the future, to be extra cautious of the potential effects that intermittent fasting can have on their fertility.

Studies on rats have found that fasting can lead to a decrease in the size of the ovaries, though other studies have found that a calorie restrictive diet with some of the same effects as intermittent fasting, can prevent some of the age-related decline in the health of eggs in female mice. There have been few human studies of the effect fasting has on fertility through studies of women who were subjected to prolonged famine or WWII captivity in concentration camps. At starvation level amounts of food for months at a time, they found that their menstrual cycle was more likely to be irregular compared to women who ate normally. This being said, they found little evidence that this affected their fertility as their ultimate family size was within average norms.

With the science so unclear, at least at the moment, the best thing for women who want to have children and try intermittent fasting to do is to be extra vigilant when it comes to the possible reproductive system side effects. Pay attention to any changes to your menstrual cycle while practicing intermittent fasting and pull back should it become irregular and especially if it discontinues. Some women have found an occasional fasting day, where they eat only 500 calories, added less stress to their cycle than a daily 16:8 or even 14:10 intermittent fasting method.

Intermittent Fasting for Moms

Fitting intermittent fasting into the life of a busy mother comes with a couple of specific issues. Getting the kids fed when you are not eating or eating very little can lead to issues of temptation that can cause an intermittent fast to fail. Children, as much as you love them, can also add a great deal of stress to your life that can contribute to some of the negative issues specific to women discussed in chapter 1.

A 16:8 or 14:10 method of intermittent fasting is likely the best version for most mothers with the eating window starting the early afternoon. This would mean skipping breakfast while you get the kids fed and allows for eating as you normally would for lunch and dinner, with slightly larger portions. Fast days can be extra difficult when dealing with feeding the kids. Cooking dinner when you are trying to eat only 500 calories on that day can be a monster of temptation, even getting takeout for the kids and being in the same room while eating your tiny fast day meal can lead to temptation issues. The smell of a pizza, when you have barely eaten during the day, will put your hunger into overdrive, doubly so if you are early in your intermittent fasting. The short daily fasts of 16:8 and 14:10, remove these issues.

(Over) Working Women, students, and intermittent fasting

Most women would agree that you don't need to have children to be stressed and tempted to break your diet. Working mothers, doubly so! The workplace provides its own pitfalls and issues when it comes to intermittent fasting. As anyone who has worked an office job knows, there can be a lot of different foods available in the office to temp those trying to fast. On the other hand, the mental benefits of intermittent fasting can be a boon for many workers. Those women with more physical jobs can also have issues with energy levels when practicing intermittent fasting, though these are more common at the start of the fast.

For overworking women with physical jobs, moving into intermittent fasting slowly and adopting a low carb diet beforehand can minimize the physical strain fasting can bring. A low carb diet often comes with a general boost in energy and alertness. Switching to such a diet before trying intermittent fasting will hopefully provide that boost that will enable your intermittent fast to succeed. Timing the initial fasting days so that you are not fasting on days that your job requires particularly heavy exertion can also help.

For office workers, a short daily fast, like the 16:8 or 14:10 can be useful when food is available in the office. If you are using a more extreme intermitting fasting method that includes very low-calorie fasting days or no-calorie fasting days, make sure to not time them on days you know the office will be full of food. Birthdays or potlucks are not great days to try and fast at the office.

Students should remember from chapter one that a benefit of the fast is an increase in mental acuity. This might have been an evolutionary tool to enable our hungry ancestors to have the brain functioning at its highest level when they needed to find food, but today, it can be strategically used to make sure your mind is at its best when you need it to be. Taking a test on a fast day might give you the edge you need for a better grade. This isn't a foolproof plan though. Sometimes, hunger can be such a distraction that it can negate the effect.

The daily fasts of 16:8 can fit into a college schedule quite well. Often meal plans will provide only two meals a day so skipping breakfast and eating lunch and dinner in the dining halls is a common eating method for college students. If your dining halls are all you can eat, there will be some temptation from sugary drinks and food items, but you will be able to eat your fill in the two meals provided.

Intermittent fasting and Women over 50

After menopause, a woman's estrogen level naturally drops, and they can put on some weight, including an increase in belly fat. Intermittent fasting can help to alleviate this, and its other benefits can assist in minimizing aging. Many women find intermittent fasting helps to elevate joint pain that can be common after 50 and studies have found that alternate day fasting has had no negative effect on bone density which can be an issue with some women as they approach 60 and 70. As their reproductive system has changed, there are fewer risks of reproductive harm for post-menopausal women.

Women over 50 can use any method of intermittent

fasting that works for their own lifestyle. Both 16:8 and 5:2 have had extensive use with women over 50, so it really comes down to fit it into your lifestyle. Retired women often have the most flexibility as they are in the most control of their schedule. For working women over 50, following the guidelines in the previous section will help them navigate intermittent fasting.

Chapter 4: Diet and Meal Plans to Maximize Your Intermittent Fast

To get the most out of your intermittent fasting routine, the type of food you eat can be almost as important as the fasting periods. While intermittent fasting can work to shed the pounds with a little limit on the amount and type of food eaten, the results will be much slower going without eating the right foods. This is especially important for intermittent fasts with extremely limited eating days such as 5:2. The more filling your 500 calorie day meals are, the easier it will be to beat temptation and stick to the fast.

For women, there is also an issue with ensuring that you eat enough protein. Women tend to get less protein in their diet than men and with the metabolic changes that intermittent fasting brings about, where the body starts feeding on fatty acids instead of consumed glucose from carbohydrates, getting enough protein can make the difference between losing or maintaining lean muscle mass.

For those including exercise in their intermittent fasting routine, protein becomes extra important. While exercising, your muscles sustain damage, and the body needs protein to prepare this damage. For protein, as opposed to fat or carbohydrates, the body does not have an on-hand supply so if you are not consuming enough protein, the wear and tear on your muscles from exercise will not heal as fast and the body can even break down some muscle tissue to use those amino acids to help repair the tired muscles.

This chapter will briefly touch on several different diet plans that can be used along with intermittent fasting to bring about the greatest weight loss benefit. With the ketogenic aspect of intermittent fasting, low carb diets are quite popular with intermittent fasting, but more carb friendly and even vegetarian diets will also be looked at.

After the look at diets, the chapter will offer examples of a single day meal plan for the 16:8 method of intermittent fasts as well as for a 500-calorie fast day in the 5:2 method of intermittent fasting.

Low Carb Diets and Intermittent Fasting

Low carb diets have had a colorful and contentious history compared to more traditional diets used for weight loss. Often, they flew in the face of conventional wisdom and their proponents have faced disbelief and scorn from those in the scientific mainstream. That said, the science behind how they work show that the same mechanisms that make intermittent fasting so effective are also behind low carb diets. This makes them a synergistic pairing, practicing both could supercharge your weight loss.

The first proponent of a low carb diet was Vilhjalmur Stefansson, the noted Canadian polar explorer. In his frequent forays into the Canadian Arctic, he had many encounters with the Inuit that lived there. The Inuit, for as long as they had lived in the harsh arctic climate, ate a diet consisting almost exclusively of animal products. The short Arctic summers were the only time the Inuit had access to wild-growing plants so for seven to nine months of the year they only had animal products to eat.

Arctic sea mammals were the most important source of food for the Inuit. Walrus, seals and especially whales were their preferred food sources. A single whale could feed an Inuit village for months. They also hunted the few land animals that live so far north such as caribou and polar bears. To survive in the frigid northern waters, the sea mammals tended to have large stores of fat. Stefansson, who studied the Inuit diet, found that they got fifty percent of their calories from fat, thirty-five percent from protein and only 15 percent from carbohydrates.

Most European descended polar explorers would bring their own rations to the north with them through the dangers involved in trips so far north often led to explorers losing their supplies or being iced in during winter and running out of supplies. In a time like that Stefansson lived and ate with the Inuit where he found the diet improved his energy level. He took his findings back to the south in the early 20th century where the conventional wisdom laughed it off as so unhealthy it could cause death.

To prove his findings, Stefansson undertook a meat only diet for an entire year, while under medical supervision, showing that a human could thrive on a meat only diet.

The Atkins Diet

The most well-known proponent of low carb diets in the last 50 years was Dr. Robert Atkins. He came out with his Atkins Diet plan in the 1970s when obesity was on the rise in the US, at the same time processed food consumption was booming. The more conventional diet plans tended towards calorie restrictive low-fat diets and again laughed off the proponent of high fat and high protein diet. The Atkins diet languished in obscurity until it became a fad diet in the early 21st century. Today Atkins diet products such as shakes, bars and frozen foods can be found in most grocery stores, though those products aren't really needed to eat a low carb diet. Some medical authorities are still resistant to this diet, and long-term consequences are still unknown though research is ongoing

The Atkins diet consists of four phases. In the first phase, induction, carbohydrates are limited to 20 grams at most, except for fiber which isn't counted. Fiber is not digestible, so it has no effect on insulin. Using these 20 grams with vegetables over simple carbohydrates such as bread is advised as you can eat a plateful of low sugar vegetables instead of a single piece of bread. The first phase is intended to induce ketosis, enabling the body to start using the fatty acids in the antipode cells for fuel instead of glucose. This phase should be used for at least two weeks but could be used longer, for greater weight loss effect.

Phase 2 of the Atkins diet, balancing, is the gradual increase of carbs in the diet, focusing on vegetables, nuts, fruits and complex carbohydrates over simple carbs and sugars. As the dieter starts to reach their goal weight, the diet moves into phase three, fine-tuning. Here more carbs are added as weight loss slows and stops when you have lost the extra pounds. The final phase is maintenance where the dieter finds a balance of good carbs while still eating primarily protein and fat

Ketogenic Diet

The ketogenic diet is basically the first phase of Atkins, where you extremely limit the number of carbs eaten to remain in ketosis. This was prescribed as a method of controlling certain epileptic conditions, but as its weight loss potential was discovered, it has become popular as a diet for weight loss.

As staying in ketosis is important for this diet, some ways to determine the presence of ketones have been devised. Ketosis changes the way your breath smells adding a fruity smell with hints of nail polish remover. There are breath ketone analyzers that can be used to determine if you are in ketosis. Ketosis can also lead to stronger smelling urine, and ketosis urine strips will show if you are still in ketosis. When on a ketogenic diet, use one of these products when you change your diet or add different foods, to make sure the changes have not moved your body out of ketosis.

Paleo Diet

One of the newer diets, the Paleo diet attempts to mimic what our ancient hunter-gatherer ancestors ate and had been touched on a few times earlier in the book. This diet is not necessarily low carb as there are plenty of carbs and sugars that can be eaten while on it, but as it favors meats and seafood over grains and processed foods, it generally is a low carb diet. Beyond meat and seafood fruits, nuts and the non-starchy vegetables are allowed in most paleo diets. The foods that the paleo diet avoids are starches, all dairy, grains as well as legumes and other beans.

The paleo diet isn't just concerned about the type of food eaten but with processing as well. All processed foods are avoided in most paleo diets, and this even includes processed meats such as cured sausages and bacon. The idea behind the bacon ban is that ancient hunter-gatherers could not cure meats, but this isn't exactly true. The curing of meats with salt or fermenting through purification are some of the most ancient forms of the preservation of meat and can be seen in use by more recent hunter-gatherer societies, but I don't make the paleo diet rules.

Of course, you do not have to follow any rules that don't work for you, so if you choose a specific low carb diet, nothing is forcing you to stick to with the exact rules. Let your body be your guide. If you discover that an addition of a little bacon doesn't lead to less weight loss in your paleo diet, have a little bacon. One thing to remember about low carb diets is that when you are eating little to no vegetables and fruit you will likely need to take a vitamin supplement for vitamin C and some of the B vitamins as they are not present in meat, unless you are eating organ meat which is not in fashion for modern western eaters.

Carb Friendlier Diets and Intermittent Fasting

Some intermittent fasting proponents think that carbs are the enemy to weight loss with intermittent fasting. There is some truth to that, but what it really comes down to is the type of carbs. Carbohydrates often get lumped together, but there is a castle different reaction in your body to different types of carbohydrates. A more accurate version of 'carbs are the enemy to weight loss' adds the word simple before carbohydrates. When eating carbs as part of an intermittent fast, stick to complex carbohydrates.

Simple carbohydrates, such as sugar and refined grains, are broken down into a readily accessible energy source for the body before they are consumed. Once they hit the stomach, they get absorbed and sent off quickly into the bloodstream to feed the cells. This causes a jump in insulin that can contribute to insulin resistance and diabetes. As the body suddenly finds itself with more fuel than it needs, it stores the excess in the fat cells, leading to weight gain.

Complex Carbohydrates, on the other hand, require the body to break them down into sugars for it to power the cells. This takes time and leads to a more gradual rise in insulin and allows the body to burn them off at that time, leading to less excess fuel being stored in the fat cells. Vegetable, whole grains, legumes, and other beans are examples of more complex carbohydrates.

Using the glycemic index to determine the glycemic load of the foods you intend to eat can be an easy way to determine which carbohydrate-laden foods you should add to your diet when intermittent fasting. When it comes to vegetables, those that grow above ground are generally lower in the glycemic index than those that grow under. Roots and tubers tend to be starchier and have more sugars. With fruit, several tropical fruits like pineapple are high on the index as are dried fruits which have more sugar than the same amount of fresh fruit as their water content has been removed.

One interesting aspect of the glycemic index of certain foods is the effect of different cooking methods. Al dente pasta has a slightly lower glycemic index than fully cooked pasta. A study of basmati rice cooked in a rice cooker or the microwave found that microwave rice has a slightly lower glycemic index. This is likely because the carbs are less accessible in undercooked foods. This can be used to slightly minimize their effect on your blood sugar.

Vegetarian Diets and Intermittent Fasting

Vegetarian diets, both low carb and carb friendly can be used in conjunction with intermittent fasting. As with non-vegetarian diets, vegetarians can use the glycemic index to eat foods that will minimize the spikes in insulin caused by simple carbohydrates. Tofu, tempeh, fat heavy dairies such as yogurt and cheese, or vegan alternatives, nuts, vegetables, and avocados are great foods for the low carb vegetarian. Grains, legumes, sugars, fruits and underground growing vegetables should be avoided to remain low carb.

Example 16:8 Meal Plans

The following meal plans represent a sample day eating a with a 16:8 intermittent fast. These start the eating period at noon, though as long as you are consistent with your eating period, it can start at any time. If you need breakfast, start it earlier. Night owls might want to start theirs a bit later. To use this plan for 14:10 intermittent fasts, move the middle meal an hour later and the dinner two hours later.

Low Carb 16:8 Example

- 12:00 — First Meal: Spaghetti Squash with chicken in a garlic lemon cream sauce

- 4:00 — Second Meal: Avocado Hummus with vegetable sticks or fried zucchini chips

- 7:00 — Third meal: Salmon cakes with homemade aioli

- Snacks — Nuts, cheese and low carb veggies like celery and pepper strips as desired

Carb Friendly 16:8 Example

- 12:00 — First Meal: Chinese Chicken Salad with soy ginger dressings (including mandarin oranges, cabbage, carrots, and scallions)

- 4:00 — Second Meal: Tuna Salad Pita Sandwich

- 7:00 — Third meal: Chicken Tikka Masala served with quinoa or cauliflower rice

- Snacks — Nuts, vegetables, cheese, and a little dark chocolate

Vegetarian 16:8 Example

- 12:00 — First Meal: Spinach tomato pasta with garlic lemon cream sauce

- 4:00 — Second Meal: Roasted vegetable salad

- 7:00 — Third meal: Black Bean Chili

- Snacks — Nuts, yogurt, roasted chickpeas as desired

Example 5:2 Fast Day Meal Plans

For 5:2 fast days, when you are limited to 500 calories a day, look to foods high in fiber to provide the most filling foods and beat hunger, especially in your first couple of fast days. Stay hydrated as well, drinking plenty of water and unsweetened tea or coffee. For the examples, the 16:8 method is followed here as well as the 5:2 and 16:8 method often go hand in hand and fasting until noon is generally pretty easy when you are already in the habit of it, making the 5:2 fast day easier to accomplish.

Low Carb 5:2 Fast Day Example

- 12:00 — First Meal: Chicken Mole with cauliflower rice (250 calories)

- 6:00 — Second Meal: Spicy carrot and lentil soup (250 calories)

- Snacks — Celery and pepper strips as well as savory, low sodium, broths

Carb Friendly 5:2 Fast Day Example

- 12:00 — First Meal: Hummus with vegetable sticks (200 calories)

- 6:00 — Second Meal: Turkey burger with corn on the cob (300 calories)

- Snacks — Celery and pepper strips as well as savory, low sodium, broths

Vegetarian 5:2 Fast Day Example

- 12:00 — First Meal: Mushroom miso soup (200 calories)

- 6:00 — Second Meal: Quinoa bowl with mushrooms and peppers (300 calories)

- Snacks — Celery and pepper strips as well as miso soup

Cheat Days:

Everyone who diets loves the idea of a cheat day, and there can actually be some benefit to one with intermittent fasting. A weekly, or biweekly, cheat day can help to stave off temptation during the rest of the week. There is also some scientific evidence that points to cheat days as a good thing. When your body burns fat to fuel its cells, the level of leptin in the fat cells falls. This can lead to the metabolism slowing, taking away some of the effectiveness of the diet. A cheat day brings those levels back up.

When scheduling a cheat day, it is most effective

with intermittent diets that have fast days where the cheat day is right before the fast. The excess calories consumed on the cheat day will hold you over during the early part of the fast day and the negative effect a cheat day can have on keeping your body burning its fat will be minimized.

Another option instead of a cheat day is to try and incorporate your temptation foods into versions that can be eaten on your specific diet. For a lot of women, chocolate is a big temptation. Not all chocolate is the same. Darker chocolates contain much less sugar than milk chocolate. Allowing for a small amount of dark chocolate in your daily diet can keep temptation at bay. Also, the cocoa powder itself has no sugar, and there are recipes available for making your own chocolate bars using calorie-free artificial sweeteners or sugar alcohols which have much less effect on blood sugar than normal sugars. Some of them can cause a laxative effect, which is stronger in some people than others, so their consumption should be moderate.

For women whose temptation is salty and crunchy, deep-fried zucchini chips can satisfy this for low carb dieters. Roasted chickpeas are another option for the crunch that can be eaten in both low carb and carb friendly diets. Seaweed or kale crisps are other options for a crunchy snack to have outside of cheat days.

Chapter 5: Role of Exercise in Intermittent Fasting

The role exercise plays in intermittent fasting can be contentious. Some proponents worry that exercise, while fasting can lead to muscle loss as the body, starved of new sources of food, will start breaking down protein to feed the working muscles. This would lead to muscle loss instead of fat. Others, particularly bodybuilders, use intermittent fasting and weight lifting to cut the fat while building bigger muscles. The truth is that for most people Intermittent fasting can shed the pounds without vigorous exercise, but exercise can help keep insulin levels in check as well as lead to more weight loss while boosting the other health benefits that intermittent fasting can provide.

This chapter will explore the best ways to include exercise in your intermittent fasting regime should you decide to include it. This will be focused on proven ways that women can exercise while minimizing the hazards specific to them with intermittent fasting. As with everything else, it is important to watch for any of the negative changes described earlier and change your fasting routine if they arise.

Do You Need to Exercise While Intermittent Fasting?

The dirty little secret that your local gym doesn't want you to know is that when it comes to weight loss, what and how you eat is 80-90 percent of the solution. The standard line that you need to burn more calories than you consume to lose weight is true, but the number of calories, or their type, are much more important than exercise. This is not to say there is no role for exercise, just that if you have not been exercising, you don't need to start just yet.

In fact, if walking back and forth to your car a few times a day is your current level of exercise, it might be best to wait until your body has adapted to intermittent fasting before adding an exercise component. This will prevent adding even more stress to your body in your initial foray into intermittent fasting. Plus, when you add exercise at a later point, you will have the energy-boosting benefit of intermittent fasting to help make exercise a bit easier.

How and When to Exercise While Intermittent Fasting.

When introducing exercise to your intermittent

fasting routine, care must be taken as to when in the fast you exercise as well as to the types of exercises you do. With a little planning ahead, your exercise routine will work with the fasting instead of against it.

As discussed in chapter two, the cells of the body want to burn glucose unless there is not enough to go around. The liver produces glycogen, a form of glucose, from some consumed nutrients or the conversion of fatty acids in the fat cells or protein in the muscle cells, when starved for other sources. When exercising the muscles will crave glucose as they burn through their available energy. Exercise while fasting can lead to the liver producing glycogen to replace its store of it. The consequences of this could be the conversion of muscle cells back into amino acids and then glucagon. This causes muscle loss.

There are two ways to prevent this. First, a low carb,

ketogenic, diet will place the liver in ketosis, enabling most cells of the body to burn the fatty acids instead of glucose or glycogen during exercise. As long as there is a good source of fatty acids stored in the fat cells, your muscles will burn it instead of your muscles. The other option, though both can be used simultaneously, is to perform your vigorous exercises when your body has enough energy from food for the muscles to use. A meal high in complex carbohydrates, if you are not going low carb, the night before your big exercise day can provide your muscles the fuel they need without cannibalizing themselves. For those choosing to go low carb, a high protein meal several hours before vigorous exercise can have the same effect.

While in your fast periods, if you want to exercise, keep it low impact. Yoga, Tai Chi, relaxed walks, etc., are all examples of lower impact exercises that can be done while on your fast periods. Listen to what your body is telling you when you exercise.

This is important for all exercise while intermittent fasting, but of extra importance for any exercise done on fasting days. Also, of utmost importance on fasting days is remaining hydrated. Drink plenty of water while you work out.

For those who have an existing exercise routine in place before starting your intermittent fasts, it is likely fine to continue this, at least on the days you are not fasting. If you are doing a daily fast such as 16:8, try to move your workouts to during your eating window or after it to exercise when your body has fuel from consumed food. If doing a 5:2 intermittent fast, go easy on your fasting days. For example, if you jog a few miles each day, take a shorter walk on your fast days, at least until your body is more adapted to the intermittent fasting.

Body Building Tips for Intermittent Fasting

Bodybuilding is not generally an exercise goal for most women, but intermittent fasting and bodybuilding often go hand in hand, so a few tips are warranted for those women who want to bulk up. Unlike using intermittent fasting for weight loss, using it to build bigger muscles requires a surplus of calories, with protein being the preferred type.

Intermittent fasting methods using short daily fasts with large eating windows each day, such as 16:8 or even the Warrior Diet with its 20:4 are preferred over methods that contain fast days. Regardless of method, keep your vigorous lifting to times when you are eating fully. Because of the calorie surplus required, your meals in the eating window will need to be larger than normal to build your muscles. As with all exercise while intermittent fasting, listen to your body and take it easy if you need.

Chapter 6: Roadmaps for Intermittent Fasting

With the information presented in the previous chapters in hand, it is time to start your first intermittent fast. This chapter will provide roadmaps that can be used to approach your intermittent fast, starting by introducing short fasts and then gradually extending and adding fasts until you are taking complete advantage of the benefits intermittent fasting can provide.

Two basic roadmaps will be discussed. One that works best with short daily fasts such as 16:8 and 14:10 with another that works better for the full day low calorie or no calorie fasts like the 5:2 and Eat Stop Eat method. As previously discussed these can be used together, for maximum benefit. For those who want to try them together, begin with the following instructions for the short daily fasts. Once you reached the level of doing the 16:8 or 14:10 on a daily basis, move on to the instructions to gradually add a low or no calorie fasting day.

Roadmap for 16:8 and 14:10 Fasts

In the weeks before you begin your initial fast, there are a few decisions you need to make. The first of these is what kind of diet you intend to follow. Are you going to go low carb or carb friendly? If you want to go low carb and are not already on a low carb diet, start following your chosen low carb diet and maintain it for at least two weeks before starting your first fast. If you intend to keep eating carbs, start to favor the carbs on the lower end of the glycemic index, avoiding processed foods and sugars.

In the weeks before you begin your initial fast, there are a few decisions you need to make. The first of these is what kind of diet you intend to follow. Are you going to go low carb or carb friendly? If you want to go low carb and are not already on a low carb diet, start following your chosen low carb diet and maintain it for at least two weeks before starting your first fast. If you intend to keep eating carbs, start to favor the carbs on the lower end of the glycemic index, avoiding processed foods and sugars.

The next decision you need to make are the days of the week you want to start fasting on. In this gradual approach, you will begin by only doing the 16:8 or 14:10 fast on two days a week. These days should be at least a day apart. For the purpose of the roadmap, Tuesday and Thursday will be used. These days were chosen based on the average

Monday through Friday work week. Starting a fast, even a gradual one, on a Monday can be extra stressful coming off of the weekend. You will need to determine for yourself which two days to start your fast.

This roadmap will be using the 16:8 schedule. If you decide for the 14:10 method, move the first meal from 'afternoon' to 'after 11 AM' and the final meal from 'before 8 PM' to 'before 9 PM.' Again, some people prefer an earlier eating window. If you want an earlier window just calculate the 8- or 10-hour eating window from your first meal. For example, if you eat breakfast at 8 in the morning, for 16:8 your last meal should be before 3 PM and for 14:10 your last meal should be before 5 PM.

First Two Weeks of the 16:8 Fast

On Sunday and Monday of your first week on the intermittent fast, eat as you normally would according to your chosen diet, eating a slightly larger meal on Monday night.

Tuesday, skip breakfast and eat a large lunch after noon and regular dinner before 8 PM. Make sure to stay hydrated in the morning but avoid all sweetened drinks before noon. Snack when hungry in the afternoon and early evening but try to skip any post 8 PM snacks or sweetened beverages.

Wednesday, eat normally according to your diet, with a slightly larger dinner before 8 PM with no snacking after dinner.

Thursday, skip breakfast again. Have a larger lunch after noon and a regular sized dinner before 8. Keep snacking limited to the afternoon and early evening, avoiding the late-night snacks or sweetened drinks. Keep hydrated in the morning with unsweetened beverages.

For Friday and through the weekend, eat normally according to your diet.

Repeat the same pattern for week two, this time without any late-night snacking on the nights before your fast days. If you find yourself suffering any of the potential negative effects discussed in the first chapter, pull back from your fast and remain at a level without the effects for a few more weeks before moving on to the next step

Week Three and Four of the 16:8 Fast

These weeks will introduce a third fasting day. It is still best to split the fasting days so that a non-fasting day is between them. You can keep the Tuesday and Thursday fasts while adding a Saturday or Sunday fast. Alternatively, you can shift your fasts to Monday, Wednesday, Friday. The choice is yours. For the purpose of the roadmap, we will be adding a Saturday fast.

Monday through Friday, follow the above instructions for the first two weeks. Eat as you normally would according to your diet on Monday, Wednesday, and Friday while skipping breakfast and any late-night snacks on Tuesday and Thursday.

Skip breakfast on Saturday, only eating between noon and 8 PM then eat normally on Sunday.

Repeat this schedule for the fourth week. By now, you should be acclimated to skipping breakfast and late-night snacks so your hunger in those shot fasts will be less than in your first week. Again, if you find the additional days adding too much stress and find you are suffering from any of the negative effects discussed in the first chapter, pull back and wait a couple of weeks before adding the extra days and moving on.

Week 5 and On

In week five, you will add a fourth fast day to your week. This day will have to be next to another fasting day. Try to choose the day that will cause the least amount of stress. If you are fasting on Tuesday, Thursday and Saturday, adding a Wednesday or Sunday fast will often work the best.

Week six introduces a fifth fasting day, with week seven adding a sixth week and week eight adding the last day of the week to the fast. Pay attention to your body as you move into a 7 day 16:8 fasting routine. As you moved into this gradually, the chances of negative side effects are low, but everyone is different, so there is no guarantee. You can stick with this amount of fasting, or once you have a handle of the 16:8, you can move on to adding an occasional longer fast.

If you have decided to go with a 14:10, once you have reached the point where you are doing it daily, gradually moving inept a 16:8 should be easy. Start slowly by switching two of your 14:10 days into 16:8. Tuesday and Thursday work well for this. After a week of that, add another and continue each week until you are eating 16:8 every day.

Moving into Longer Fasts

Pick the least stressful day to start a longer fast but try not to use a day where boredom could be an issue as it often leads to temptation. Eat an extra-large meal the night before and make sure to keep hydrated during the day.

The next step depends on the type of fast you want to use. For a no-calorie fast, after the large meal the night before, skip your lunch and have a late afternoon snack and dinner as you normally would. Next week, skip the afternoon snack and eat a big dinner. If your goal is to follow an eat stop eat routine, you have reached it.

If you want to get to an entire fasting day, continue on. With the third week, reduce the size of the large dinner to a normal sized dinner. Reducing the size of the dinner again the next week to a light, filling meal the next week will get you ready for going an entire day without food. You can take this further by moving towards an alternative day fast by slowly following the gradual reduction for another day of the week, continuing until you are eating only every other day.

Be warned that this is an extreme fast that is not for everyone. Be wary of the potential negative side effects when trying this sort of fast. They are much more likely with an extreme fast.

If you decide to try a low calorie fast, the method is much less extreme. Like before, you will be adding one a week to start and can move up to two if you prefer. For the first week, eat a large meal the night before and then restricts the size of your lunch by about half as normal. Eat normally the rest of the day. Next week, eat the half size lunch but limit your afternoon snacking to low-calorie options. Vegetable sticks and miso soup would work. The following week eat a half size lunch, low-calorie snacks and reduce the size of your dinner by half. Over the next two weeks reduce your lunch and then your dinner in half and you will have a low-calorie fast day. You can add another, using the same gradual plan to bring your intermittent fasting into 5:2.

Again, this fast isn't for everyone, so do not fret if you prefer a less extreme fast. Keep paying attention to your body and watch for negative side effects.

Chapter 7: Mindset and Motivation

As I mentioned in my introduction, I have tried and failed at many diets. The thing I failed to mention is that there's absolutely nothing wrong with that! It's perfectly normal for you to go through some trial and error when trying to figure out what works best for your body.

Let's think about the science of diet and nutrition for a moment. Let's say that a scientist has come up with a theory for the most perfect diet. They know the exact number of calories, carbs, fat, fiber, and other nutrients that someone should have throughout their life in order to keep weight off, increase muscle mass and have healthy blood.

Now, how is this scientist supposed to test this diet to see if it works? First, they would have to find a group of babies and make sure that each baby ate the exact same meals from birth until about the age of 18. Although that seems nearly impossible, let's just pretend for a moment that it could be done. Even if we could get a group of babies to eat the exact same meals for their entire childhood, it doesn't end there now, does it? Because our health is also related to how much we exercise and how much daily movement we get. So the test babies would not only have to eat the exact same meals and snacks for 18 years, but they would also have to do the same activities and daily workout routines. If you were hopeful before, surely now you can see that this kind of experiment is impossible.

Even if the experiment could be done, it doesn't take into account the genetic makeup of the individuals. Some of them may have a history of diabetes in their family, others may have a history of heart disease. Even if you did take these into account when testing the diet, the diet could turn out to be "perfect' for people who have a history of heart disease but not perfect for people who have a history of diabetes. Now the "perfect diet" isn't perfect for everyone so it's just like any of the diets we have today. Everyone is different so we all have different needs, there is no one size fits all.

This is why it is *so important* for you to always listen to your body and to not beat yourself up if you make mistakes.

My experience with Intermittent Fasting

Just like any new lifestyle, IF came with its challenges at first. I would have the regular cravings, miss the snacking before bed and wish that I could eat a delicious brunch on Sunday mornings with my boyfriend. All that being said, this lifestyle was the easiest diet-related change I have ever made in my life.

Most diets restrict the foods you eat and I find that it makes me crave those foods even more. It's like telling a child that he can't have candy, but if you hadn't said the word candy in the first place, he never would have wanted it. With this diet, all I have to do is makes sure I eat around noon and have dinner before 8 pm. It's really easy now but at first, it felt impossible.

My best advice for getting around the hurdles is to start slow and listen to your body. Remember that eating and hunger are habitual. If your body is used to waking up and then eating breakfast, it is going to feel hungry when you don't give it breakfast at the time it is used to. This is why you should wean yourself off of breakfast by having a lighter meal, then just a snack, then just some coffee and eventually just water.

Since I was so determined to make this work, I often found myself pushing too hard and trying to get results too quickly. I would starve myself, feel super hungry and go without food until I felt like fainting. This is not the way you want to introduce this diet to your system. If you are doing it correctly, you shouldn't ever feel starved or like you are going to pass out. By the time you are down to only 2 or 3 meals within an 8-hour window, your body should be totally used to it and it shouldn't make you feel sick or void of energy.

Once I finally got this diet to work and was down to only three meals within an 8-hour window, I started seeing results. I am only 5'3 and went from 135 lbs to 120 lbs in a few months. After that I didn't lose any weight but noticed my muscle mass was increasing and it was a lot easier for me to complete more complicated weightlifting workouts. Since then I have focused on bodybuilding and weightlifting competitions. My body looks toned and muscular, but I don't have the big bulk that I would if I was doing things unnaturally.

My favorite part of IF is that it's all natural and you're using your bodies own hormones in order to get the results you want. It has made me so proud of my body because I look healthy, fit and feel very strong without looking like I'm a man with a woman's head on my body. I have also noticed an increase in endurance so I am able to run and do cardio workouts for much longer periods of time.

Always be proud of yourself, it's ok to make mistakes

Intermittent fasting is a simple diet to add to your

lifestyle. It is very forgiving of cheat days so definitely use those cheat days when you just can't resist or if you're at a party or other social outing. Remember that keeping up a healthy lifestyle just means that your daily routine is healthy, it doesn't mean that you can never spend a day enjoying yourself.

I like to look at it this way. If every day you are eating chips after dinner, donuts for breakfast and having soda instead of water, you don't deserve to eat a piece of cake at your best friend's birthday party! But, if you eat healthy, well-balanced meals, often give your body a break from food so it can detox and strive to keep a healthy exercise plan on a weekly basis – you go ahead and gobble that piece of cake up!

One little piece of cake or another kind of treat is not going to throw everything off. Don't be so hard on yourself. Remember that your body is very forgiving and can take a lot of abuse before it starts to go downhill. If your daily routine is generally a healthy one, be proud of yourself for keeping it up.

The craving substitutes

I mentioned before that when I restrict myself from eating yummy treats, I often find myself craving them more than I would if I didn't even put the restriction on myself. One way to combat this is to avoid temptation. Keep unhealthy snacks or treats out of the house so that they are not so easily accessible. This way, if you find yourself craving some ice cream, you would actually have to get up, walk to the store and buy some. It's a lot more effort and if you go through that effort, you're a lot more deserving of it than if you just walked to the freezer!

What I like to do is substitute my cravings for

something healthier. In the example above, I mentioned a craving for ice cream. Rather than going to the store and getting a tub of ice cream to sit in my freezer, I may just go down to the convenience store and grab a small popsicle that is less than a 100 calories. Or I might grab a small cup of frozen yogurt. Even better is making a healthy smoothie at home and freezing it for when that ice cream craving comes along.

Here are some healthy foods that you can use to satisfy your unhealthy cravings:

- Chips: Rice cake chips with your favorite flavoring or popcorn
- Candy: Chocolate dipped nuts, dried fruit
- Milk chocolate: Dark Chocolate
- Soda: Flavored water, carbonated water
- Frozen treats: Frozen grapes, frozen yogurt or homemade smoothies

Keep moving forward

As a final note, I just want to say that you should never beat yourself up for slipping or giving in to a craving. Life moves forward, and so should you. Don't dwell on mistakes or slip-ups that you've made in the past, and absolutely do not try to use today to make up for yesterday's mistakes.

Let me explain what I mean by that. If you are trying to start fasting, you might find yourself hungry at 9:00 pm (outside of your eating window). So you give in and have a snack. This does not mean that you should try to make up for this mistake by eating later the following day!

Mistakes happen and if it happens to you, just eat a snack and start the next day fresh. The reason for this is that if you constantly try to make up for yesterday's mistakes, you will be playing a constant game of catch up that will leave you starving and frustrated. Each day should be looked at separately. So if you start your eating window at noon on most days but slipped up the night before, do not change the noon start date. Just try it again until your body gets used to it.

I'm sorry to keep saying this but I'm going to repeat this one more time: when learning how to fast – you should never be starving to the point where you feel like you're going to faint! A little bit of hunger is ok but too much and you're just going to get frustrated and give up. It's ok to give in to the hunger pains while you're teaching your body something new.

While we're on the topic of looking forward - don't check your results right away by constantly looking at your tummy in the mirror. Instead, focus on eating at the right time, drinking lots of water and getting your body used to a new lifestyle. Then one day you'll start to see results and you'll be proud of all the hard work that you've put in. The results don't happen by hating yourself in front of the mirror, they happen by being proud of yourself and making little decisions throughout the day.

Your FREE Intermittent Fasting Meal Plan

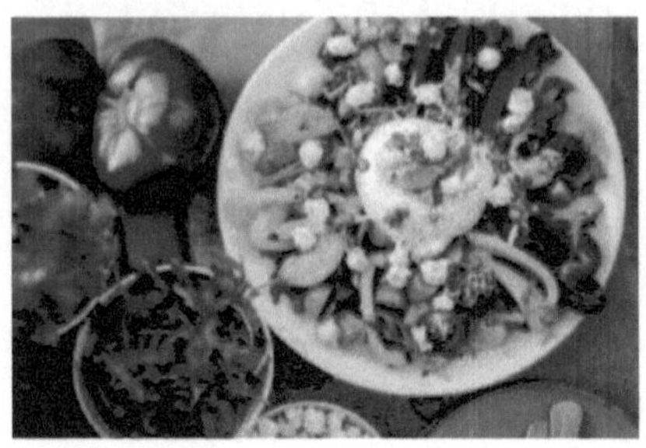

Subscribe to my email list and get your free IF meal plan and food guide. Learn what foods to avoid and what foods to stick to during time-restricted eating.

Visit:

HannahGoldenLifestyle.com/fastingmealplan

Conclusion

Thank you for making it through to the end of *Intermittent Fasting for Women,* and I hope this is the beginning of a new healthy lifestyle for you. Remember that introducing a new lifestyle or diet plan to your body can be tough at first but keep at it and you'll start seeing results in no time. I don't want to promise you the moon here, but science and countless people who have tried this lifestyle can say that the odds are definitely in your favor.

Because you are a woman, intermittent fasting presents risks and side effects that you wouldn't experience if you were a man. It is for this reason that you should be extra vigilant when starting this lifestyle and introduce it slowly so that it is not a shock to your system. As a woman, you can definitely experience the benefits and positive effects of IF but it must be done in a safe and healthy way.

Finally, if you found this book useful in any way, a review on Amazon is always appreciated!

Your FREE Intermittent Fasting Meal Plan

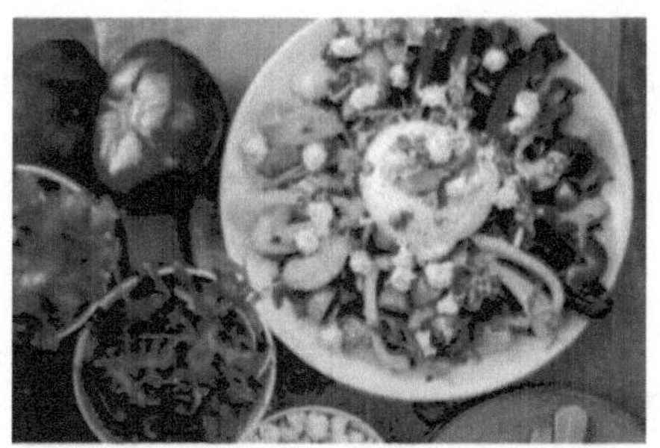

Subscribe to my email list and get your free IF meal plan and food guide. Learn what foods to avoid and what foods to stick to during time-restricted eating.

Visit:

HannahGoldenLifestyle.com/fastingmealplan